STRENGTH CONFIDENCE AND RESILIENCE

Harnessing the power of exercise to build strength and unlocking the potential for building confidence and resilience in woman empowering them to thrive and live a healthy lifestyle

BOBBY CARL

TABLE OF CONTENT

INTRODUCTION

INTRODUCTION

In the realm of fitness, myths surrounding strength training for women persist, often deterring them from reaping the numerous benefits this form of exercise offers. It's time to debunk these misconceptions and empower women to embrace strength training as an integral part of their fitness journey.

Unmasking Myths: Strength Training for Women Strength training for women has evolved from being a niche activity to a cornerstone of fitness regimens worldwide. Historically, there existed a misconception that weightlifting or strength training was exclusively for men, fearing bulky muscles or compromising femininity. However, modern understanding and research have debunked these myths, revealing the profound benefits of strength exercises tailored to women.

The strength training for women represents a pivotal shift in the fitness landscape, emphasizing empowerment, resilience, and holistic health. Unlike traditional cardio-focused routines, strength training offers a myriad of advantages specifically beneficial for women. It enhances bone density, reducing the risk of osteoporosis, a condition more prevalent among females. Moreover, it promotes lean muscle mass, which not only boosts metabolism but also fosters a toned physique.

Beyond physical changes, engaging in strength exercises fosters mental fortitude and confidence, breaking societal norms and stereotypes. Women of all ages and fitness levels can partake in strength training, customizing routines to suit individual goals and preferences. From free weights to bodyweight exercises and resistance bands, the options are diverse, ensuring inclusivity and accessibility.

In essence, the strength exercises for women signifies a paradigm shift towards embracing strength, resilience, and self-confidence, revolutionizing fitness culture and empowering women to unlock their full potential, both physically and mentally.

In the realm of fitness, myths surrounding strength training for women persist, often deterring them from reaping the numerous benefits this form of exercise offers. It's time to debunk these misconceptions and empower women to embrace strength training as an integral part of their fitness journey.

SOME OF THE MYTH SURROUNDING WOMAN STRENGTH TRAINING

✓ *Myth: Strength Training Will Make Women Bulky:* *Reality:* One of the most common misconceptions is that lifting weights will result in a bulky physique. In truth, women typically lack the testosterone levels needed to develop significant muscle mass. Strength training, instead, enhances muscle tone, leading to a lean and sculpted appearance.

✓ *Myth: Cardio is the Only Way for Women to Stay Fit:* *Reality:* While cardio has its benefits, an exclusive focus on cardiovascular exercise neglects the advantages of strength training. Combining both forms of exercise creates a well-rounded fitness routine, promoting overall health, and enhancing weight management.

✓ *Myth: Women Should Stick to Light Weights and High Reps:* *Reality:* Women can benefit from lifting heavier weights and incorporating lower rep ranges. This approach promotes strength gains without necessarily increasing muscle size, fostering a balanced and effective workout routine.

✓ *Myth: Strength Training is Unsafe for Joints and Bones:*
Reality: When performed with proper form, strength training is not only safe but also beneficial for joint and bone health. Weight-bearing exercises contribute to improved bone density, reducing the risk of osteoporosis, especially crucial for women as they age.

✓ *Myth: Women Should Avoid Strength Training During Pregnancy:*
Reality: In many cases, strength training can be safe and beneficial during pregnancy. However, it's essential to consult with a healthcare professional and modify exercises as necessary. Properly adapted strength training routines can help maintain fitness levels and prepare the body for childbirth.

✓ *Myth: You Need a Gym Membership for Effective Strength Training:*
Reality: Strength training doesn't always require a gym membership. Bodyweight exercises, resistance bands, and simple home equipment can be effective tools for building strength. Women can tailor their workouts to their preferences and availability of resources.

✓ ***Myth: Older Women Should Avoid Strength Training:***
Reality*:* Strength training becomes increasingly important as women age. It helps counteract muscle loss, maintain bone density, and enhance overall functional fitness. Older women can adapt strength training routines to suit their abilities and needs.

✓ ***Myth: Women Will Get Weaker if They Stop Strength Training:***
Reality*:* The notion that strength gained through training will rapidly diminish is unfounded. While consistency is key, taking breaks or modifying routines doesn't automatically lead to significant strength loss. Regular activity helps maintain strength over time.

By dispelling these myths surrounding strength training for women, we encourage a shift in perspective. Strength training emerges not as an intimidating or unsuitable pursuit for women but as a versatile and empowering tool for achieving holistic health and fitness goals. It's time for women to embrace the benefits of strength training, redefine stereotypes, and confidently navigate their fitness journeys.

CHAPTER ONE

Metabolism, often referred to as the body's 'internal engine,' plays a pivotal role in our overall health and well-being. The concept of an improved metabolism has sparked interest among those seeking to enhance energy levels, manage weight, and promote overall vitality.

Metabolism encompasses all the biochemical processes that occur within the body to maintain life. It involves two main components:

BMR represents the calories your body requires at rest to maintain basic physiological functions such as breathing, circulation, and cell production. It constitutes a significant portion of your daily energy expenditure.

Physical Activity and Thermic Effect of Food (TEF)

CHAPTER ONE

The Science Behind Improved Metabolism

Metabolism, often referred to as the body's internal engine, plays a pivotal role in our overall health and well-being. The concept of an improved metabolism has sparked interest among those seeking to enhance energy levels, manage weight, and promote overall vitality

Understanding Metabolism:

Metabolism encompasses all the biochemical processes that occur within the body to maintain life. It involves two main components:

Basal Metabolic Rate (BMR):

BMR represents the calories your body requires at rest to maintain basic physiological functions such as breathing, circulation, and cell production. It constitutes a significant portion of your daily energy expenditure.

Physical activity and thermic effect of Food (TEF):

Physical activity and TEF encompass the calories burned through exercise and the energy required to digest, absorb, and process the nutrients from the food you consume.

Methods to Improve Metabolism:

Strength Training and Muscle Mass

Engaging in regular strength training is a potent strategy to improve metabolism. Muscle tissue requires more energy at rest than fat tissue, contributing to a higher BMR. As individuals build and maintain lean muscle mass, their metabolism receives a natural boost.

High-Intensity Interval Training (HIIT):

HIIT workouts involve short bursts of intense activity followed by periods of rest or lower-intensity exercise. This approach has been shown to elevate metabolism both during and after the workout, leading to increased calorie burn throughout the day.

Adequate Protein Intake:

Consuming an adequate amount of protein is crucial for maintaining and building lean muscle mass. Protein has a higher thermic effect compared to fats and carbohydrates, meaning the body expends more energy in digesting and metabolizing protein-rich foods.

Regular Physical Activity:

Physical activity in any form contributes to an enhanced metabolism. Whether it's walking, jogging, swimming, or dancing, the key is to stay consistently active. This not only burns calories but also positively influences overall metabolic efficiency.

Proper Hydration:

Dehydration can slow down metabolism. Drinking an ample amount of water supports various metabolic processes, including nutrient transport and the breakdown of stored energy.

Adequate Sleep:

Quality sleep is essential for metabolic health. Sleep deprivation can disrupt hormonal balance, leading to increased hunger and a slower metabolism. Aim for 7-9 hours of quality sleep each night.

Spice Up Your Meals:

Certain spices, such as cayenne pepper, contain compounds that may temporarily boost metabolism by increasing body temperature. While the effect is modest, incorporating these spices into meals can add a flavorful kick to your metabolism.

Improving metabolism is not a mysterious or elusive goal; it's a science-backed journey that involves lifestyle choices and habits.

By incorporating strength training, embracing a variety of physical activities, maintaining a balanced diet with sufficient protein, staying hydrated, prioritizing sleep, and adding a dash of spice to your meals, you can stoke the metabolic fire within. Remember, the key lies in sustainable practices that support your overall health and vitality.

How strength training boosts metabolic rate.

Strength training is a powerful tool for boosting metabolic rate, and this effect is attributed to several physiological mechanisms. Understanding these mechanisms sheds light on why incorporating strength training into a fitness routine is beneficial for those looking to enhance metabolism and manage weight. Here's how strength training influences metabolic rate:

Increased Lean Muscle Mass:

One of the primary ways strength training impacts metabolism is by increasing lean muscle mass. Muscles are metabolically active tissues, meaning they require energy (calories) for maintenance and function. When you engage in regular strength training, you stimulate the growth and maintenance of muscle tissue.

Elevated Resting Metabolic Rate (RMR):

Resting Metabolic Rate (RMR) refers to the number of calories your body needs at rest to maintain basic physiological functions such as breathing, circulation, and cell production. Lean muscle mass contributes significantly to RMR because muscle tissue demands more energy compared to fat tissue. As you build and maintain muscle through strength training, your RMR increases, leading to a higher baseline calorie expenditure even when you are at rest.

After-burn Effect (Excess Post-Exercise Oxygen Consumption - EPOC):

Intense strength training sessions can lead to an increased oxygen debt, which the body needs to repay after the workout. This post-exercise oxygen consumption, or after-burn effect, results in additional calories being burned in the hours following a strength training session. The body expends energy to restore oxygen levels, repair tissues, and replenish energy stores, contributing to an extended calorie-burning period.

Metabolic Adaptations:

Strength training can prompt metabolic adaptations that enhance energy expenditure. This includes improvements in insulin sensitivity and the body's ability to utilize nutrients more efficiently. These adaptations contribute to a more favorable metabolic profile, promoting better overall metabolic health.

Caloric Burn during Exercise:

While the impact of the actual exercise session on total daily caloric expenditure might be smaller compared to cardiovascular activities like running or cycling, strength training still burns calories during the workout. The cumulative effect of consistent strength training sessions contributes to overall calorie expenditure.

Prevention of Age-Related Muscle Loss:

As individuals age, there's a natural tendency to lose muscle mass, which can lead to a decline in metabolic rate. Strength training is particularly crucial for older adults as it helps counteract age-related muscle loss, preserving or even increasing muscle mass and, consequently, maintaining a higher metabolic rate.

In conclusion, strength training influences metabolic rate by fostering the growth and maintenance of lean muscle mass, elevating resting metabolic rate, inducing the afterburn effect, and promoting metabolic adaptations. Including a well-rounded strength training routine in your fitness regimen not only contributes to a more sculpted physique but also acts as a dynamic strategy for enhancing overall metabolic health and supporting weight management goals.

The long-term impact on weight management and fat loss.

The long-term impact of strength training on weight management and fat loss is substantial, making it a crucial component of a comprehensive and sustainable approach to achieving and maintaining a healthy body composition. Here are several ways in which strength training influences weight management and fat loss over the long term:

Increased Resting Metabolic Rate (RMR):
As mentioned earlier, strength training contributes to the development and maintenance of lean muscle mass. Since muscle tissue is more metabolically active than fat tissue, an increase in muscle mass elevates Resting Metabolic Rate (RMR). This means that individuals with higher muscle mass burn more calories at rest, aiding in

weight management by creating a favorable calorie balance.

Caloric Expenditure Beyond the Workout:

The after-burn effect, scientifically known as Excess Post-Exercise Oxygen Consumption (EPOC), plays a role in long-term fat loss. After an intense strength training session, the body continues to burn calories during the recovery and repair processes, contributing to an extended period of elevated caloric expenditure. This post-exercise effect can support weight management efforts over time.

Improved Insulin Sensitivity:

Strength training enhances insulin sensitivity, which is crucial for regulating blood sugar levels. Improved insulin sensitivity allows the body to use carbohydrates more efficiently, reducing the likelihood of excess glucose being stored as fat. This metabolic benefit is significant for long-term weight management and the prevention of insulin-related issues, such as type 2 diabetes.

Maintenance of Muscle Mass During Weight Loss:

When individuals engage in a calorie deficit for weight loss, there's a risk of losing both fat and muscle mass.

Incorporating strength training into a weight loss program helps preserve lean muscle mass. This

is crucial because maintaining muscle mass ensures that a higher percentage of the weight lost comes from fat rather than muscle, contributing to a more favorable body composition.

Enhanced Fat Oxidation:

Regular strength training has been associated with increased fat oxidation, which means the body becomes more efficient at using fat as a fuel source. This metabolic adaptation is beneficial for long-term fat loss and weight management.

Positive Impact on Body Composition:

Beyond the number on the scale, strength training positively influences body composition. As individuals gain muscle and reduce body fat, they experience a transformation in their physique. This shift toward a leaner body composition not only contributes to improved aesthetics but also supports sustainable weight management.

Sustained Metabolic Adaptations:

Over the long term, consistent engagement in strength training leads to sustained metabolic adaptations. The body becomes more efficient at utilizing nutrients, regulating energy balance, and maintaining a higher metabolic rate. These adaptations create an environment conducive to lasting fat loss and weight management.

It's important to note that while strength training plays a significant role, achieving and maintaining a healthy weight requires a comprehensive approach that includes a balanced diet, regular physical activity, and other lifestyle factors.

Incorporating strength training into this holistic strategy enhances its effectiveness, providing individuals with a sustainable and health-focused path to long-term weight management and fat loss.

CHAPTER TWO

How strength training helps in preventing osteoporosis.

Strength training is a potent ally in the prevention of osteoporosis, a condition characterized by the weakening of bones, making them fragile and more susceptible to fractures. Osteoporosis is particularly common in postmenopausal women, but it can affect both men and women of all ages. Here's how strength training plays a crucial role in maintaining bone health and preventing osteoporosis:

Bone Density Improvement:

One of the primary benefits of strength training for preventing osteoporosis is its positive impact on bone density. Weight-bearing exercises, such as strength training, stimulate bone formation by subjecting bones to mechanical stress. This stress prompts the bones to adapt by becoming denser and stronger, reducing the risk of fractures associated with osteoporosis.

Stimulation of Bone-Forming Cells:

Strength training activates osteoblasts, the cells responsible for bone formation. When you engage in weight-bearing exercises, especially those involving resistance, the mechanical loading on bones signals osteoblasts to produce more bone tissue. This process is crucial for maintaining and increasing bone density, ultimately contributing to the prevention of osteoporosis.

Prevention of Bone Loss:

As individuals age, there is a natural tendency for bone density to decrease. Strength training counteracts this by helping to prevent age-related bone loss. Regular resistance exercises create a constant demand on the skeletal system, sending signals to the body that maintaining bone mass is essential.

Promotion of Bone Remodeling:

Bone remodeling is a continuous process in the body where old bone tissue is broken down (resorption), and new bone tissue is formed (formation). Strength training contributes to this process by promoting bone remodeling. This dynamic cycle is crucial for maintaining bone strength, integrity, and preventing the onset of osteoporosis.

Specificity of Exercise:
Different types of strength training exercises can target specific areas prone to bone loss. Weight-bearing exercises that focus on the spine, hips, and wrists are particularly beneficial for preventing osteoporosis, as these areas are commonly affected by bone density reduction.

Enhancement of Muscular Strength and Balance:
In addition to its direct impact on bones, strength training improves muscular strength and balance. Strong muscles provide better support to the skeletal system and reduce the risk of falls, a significant concern for individuals with osteoporosis. Enhanced balance further diminishes the likelihood of fractures.

Adaptability for Individuals of All Ages
Strength training can be adapted to accommodate individuals of all ages and fitness levels. Whether through resistance bands, free weights, or weight machines, the intensity and complexity of strength training exercises can be adjusted to meet individual needs, making it accessible for those at various stages of life.

Consistency and Long-Term Benefits

The preventive effects of strength training against osteoporosis are most pronounced when it is part of a consistent, long-term fitness routine. Regular and ongoing engagement in strength training helps build and maintain bone density over time, providing sustained protection against osteoporosis.

In conclusion, strength training is a vital component of a comprehensive approach to bone health and the prevention of osteoporosis. Its ability to stimulate bone density improvement, promote bone remodeling, and enhance overall musculoskeletal health makes it a valuable strategy for individuals looking to maintain strong and resilient bones throughout their lives. Always consult with a healthcare professional or fitness expert before starting a new exercise program, especially if you have pre-existing conditions or concerns about bone health.

The connection between strength training and bone health.

Strength training plays a pivotal role in enhancing joint stability, contributing to improved overall joint health and functionality. Joint stability is crucial for everyday movements, sports performance, and injury prevention. Here are key ways in which strength training contributes to better joint stability:

Muscular Support:

The muscles surrounding a joint act as dynamic stabilizers. As these muscles contract and relax during strength training exercises, they provide active support to the joint, helping maintain its proper alignment and stability. Well-developed muscles contribute to joint integrity by preventing excessive movement and ensuring controlled, coordinated actions.

Increased Muscle Strength:

Strength training is designed to increase the strength of muscles, tendons, and ligaments. As the strength of these supporting structures improves, they become more capable of stabilizing joints under various loads and during dynamic movements. This increased strength contributes to a more stable foundation for joint movement.

Enhanced Proprioception:

Proprioception refers to the body's ability to sense its position in space. Strength training exercises often involve complex movements that challenge proprioception. This heightened awareness of joint position and movement contributes to improved joint stability. Individuals who engage in strength training develop a better sense of how their joints are positioned, reducing the risk of injuries caused by misalignment.

Improved Balance and Coordination:

Strength training exercises often require coordinated movements that engage multiple muscle groups simultaneously. This type of training improves overall balance and coordination, essential components of joint stability. Enhanced balance ensures that the body can distribute forces evenly, reducing the likelihood of joint instability or injury.

Joint-Specific Training:

Tailoring strength training exercises to target specific joints is a common practice. For example, exercises like leg presses and squats target the knee joint, while shoulder presses and lateral raises focus on the shoulder joint. Joint-specific training allows for the development of the muscles and structures directly responsible for stabilizing a particular joint.

Prevention of Muscle Imbalances:

Strength training helps prevent muscle imbalances, a common cause of joint instability. When certain muscle groups are significantly stronger than their opposing counterparts, it can lead to joint misalignment. A well-balanced strength training program ensures that opposing muscle groups are equally developed, promoting joint stability.

Protection Against Overuse Injuries:

Overuse injuries often result from repetitive movements that place excessive stress on a joint. Strength training diversifies movement patterns and strengthens supporting structures, reducing the risk of overuse injuries. By enhancing joint stability, strength training helps protect joints from wear and tear associated with repetitive activities.

Adaptation to Functional Movements:

Functional movements mimic activities of daily living. Strength training that incorporates functional exercises such as squats, lunges, and rotational movements helps the body adapt to the demands of real-world activities. This adaptability contributes to improved joint stability during various functional movements.

In summary, strength training promotes better joint stability through increased muscular support, enhanced proprioception, improved balance and coordination, joint-specific training, prevention of muscle imbalances, protection against overuse injuries, and adaptation to functional movements. Integrating a well-rounded strength training program into your fitness routine can significantly contribute to joint health, reducing the risk of injuries and enhancing overall movement efficiency. Always consult with a healthcare professional or fitness expert before starting a new exercise program, especially if you have pre-existing conditions or concerns about joint health.

CHAPTER THREE

How strength training contributes to better joint stability.

Strength training plays a crucial role in maintaining flexibility and reducing the risk of injuries by addressing several key aspects of musculoskeletal health. While strength training is often associated with building muscle mass and strength, it also contributes significantly to joint mobility, flexibility, and injury prevention. Here's how strength training impacts flexibility and helps minimize the risk of injuries:

Improved Joint Range of Motion (ROM):

Strength training exercises involve a full range of motion, requiring joints to move through their complete ROM. This dynamic movement helps improve joint flexibility by stretching and strengthening the muscles and connective tissues around the joint. Over time, this contributes to increased flexibility and mobility.

Enhanced Muscle Elasticity:

Strength training, particularly when performed with a focus on controlled movements and proper form, promotes muscle elasticity. The controlled stretching and contracting of muscles during resistance exercises improve the flexibility of the muscle fibers and surrounding connective tissues. This increased muscle elasticity contributes to overall flexibility and joint range of motion.

Dynamic Stretching as Part of Warm-Up:

Many strength training programs incorporate dynamic stretching as part of the warm-up routine. Dynamic stretching involves controlled, active movements that take muscles and joints through their full range of motion. This type of stretching helps increase blood flow to the muscles, enhances flexibility, and prepares the body for the demands of the upcoming strength training session.

Prevention of Muscular Imbalances:

Muscular imbalances, where certain muscle groups are significantly stronger or tighter than others, can lead to reduced flexibility and an increased risk of injuries. Strength training programs designed with a focus on balance ensure that opposing muscle groups are equally developed, preventing imbalances and promoting overall flexibility.

Injury Prevention Through Stability:

Strength training not only improves muscle strength but also enhances joint stability. Strong, stable joints are less prone to misalignments and excessive movement that can lead to injuries. As muscles surrounding a joint become stronger, they provide better support and protection, reducing the risk of injuries during both everyday activities and more intense physical pursuits.

Functional Flexibility:

Strength training exercises that involve functional movements contribute to what is often referred to as "functional flexibility." Functional flexibility is the ability to move the body in a coordinated manner through various planes of motion, mimicking real-world activities. This type of flexibility is essential for preventing injuries during activities that require dynamic and multi-directional movements.

Adaptability to Diverse Training Modalities:

Strength training can be adapted to include various training modalities, such as resistance bands, free weights, or bodyweight exercises. This adaptability allows individuals to choose exercises that suit their preferences and address specific flexibility goals. Incorporating a variety of exercises helps ensure a well-rounded approach to flexibility training.

Including static stretching as part of the cool-down phase of a strength training session helps improve flexibility and prevent muscle tightness. Static stretching, where muscles are stretched and held in a stationary position, can help alleviate muscle tension, reduce stiffness, and enhance overall flexibility.

In conclusion, strength training is a versatile and effective tool for maintaining flexibility and reducing the risk of injuries. By incorporating dynamic stretching, preventing muscular imbalances, enhancing joint stability, and promoting functional flexibility, strength training contributes to a well-rounded approach to musculoskeletal health. Always consult with a healthcare professional or fitness expert before starting a new exercise program, especially if you have pre-existing conditions or concerns about flexibility and injury prevention.

CHAPTER FOUR

The psychological benefits of strength training, including stress reduction.

Strength training goes beyond the physical realm, offering a wealth of psychological benefits that contribute to overall well-being. Among these benefits, stress reduction is a notable outcome that has been supported by research. Here's an examination of the psychological benefits of strength training, with a focus on its stress-reducing effects:

Release of Endorphins:

Strength training, particularly high-intensity workouts, triggers the release of endorphins, often referred to as "feel-good" hormones. Endorphins act as natural mood elevators and pain relievers, creating a positive and euphoric sensation. This neurochemical response contributes to a sense of well-being and can alleviate stress and anxiety.

Reduction in Cortisol Levels:

Cortisol, often known as the stress hormone, is released in response to stress. Regular strength training has been associated with a reduction in cortisol levels. While cortisol is a necessary hormone for certain bodily functions, chronic elevation due to stress can have negative effects. Strength training helps balance cortisol levels, promoting a more resilient stress response.

Enhanced Sleep Quality:

Regular strength training has been linked to improvements in sleep quality. Quality sleep is crucial for mental health and stress management. The physical exertion and hormonal changes induced by strength training contribute to better sleep patterns, reducing the impact of stress on sleep quality.

Empowerment and Confidence:

Strength training empowers individuals by helping them achieve physical goals and milestones. As individuals witness improvements in strength, endurance, and physical appearance, they often experience a boost in confidence and self-esteem. Feeling capable and strong contributes to a positive mindset and resilience in the face of stressors.

Cognitive Benefits:

Physical exercise, including strength training, has cognitive benefits that extend beyond the body. It has been linked to improved cognitive function, including enhanced memory, attention, and problem-solving skills. A sharper mind can better cope with stress and navigate challenges effectively.

Mind-Body Connection:

Strength training fosters a strong mind-body connection. Concentrating on the proper form, controlled movements, and the mind-muscle connection during exercises encourages individuals to be present in the moment. This mindfulness can be a powerful stress-relief strategy, as it helps redirect attention away from stressors.

Sense of Accomplishment:

Achieving fitness goals in strength training, whether it's lifting heavier weights, completing more repetitions, or mastering a new exercise, provides a profound sense of accomplishment. This positive reinforcement can counteract the negative effects of stress and contribute to a more optimistic outlook.

Social Support and Community:
Strength training can be a social activity, whether individuals engage in group classes, workout with a partner, or connect with a fitness community. Social interactions and support systems play a crucial role in stress management. Sharing experiences, challenges, and successes with others fosters a sense of community and belonging.

Outlet for Frustration and Tension:
Strength training serves as a physical outlet for pent-up frustration and tension. The act of lifting weights or engaging in intense physical activity provides a healthy and constructive way to release stress and tension, promoting emotional well-being.

Long-Term Stress Resilience:
The consistent practice of strength training contributes to long-term stress resilience. Building physical and mental strength through regular workouts provides individuals with tools and coping mechanisms that extend beyond the gym, helping them navigate life's challenges with greater ease.

In summary, the psychological benefits of strength training, including stress reduction, are multifaceted. From the neurochemical effects of endorphins and cortisol regulation to the empowerment gained through physical accomplishments, strength training offers a holistic approach to mental well-being. Integrating strength training into a routine can be a powerful strategy for managing stress and promoting a positive mindset. Always consult with a healthcare professional or fitness expert before starting a new exercise program, especially if you have pre-existing conditions or concerns about stress management.

The impact of strength training on mood, cognitive function, and overall mental health

Strength training has a profound impact on various aspects of mental health, including mood, cognitive function, and overall psychological well-being. The connection between physical activity and mental health is well-established, and strength training, in particular, offers a unique set of benefits that positively influence mental and emotional well-being. Here's an exploration of how strength training affects mood, cognitive function, and overall mental health:

Mood Enhancement:

Strength training has been linked to improvements in mood, with the release of endorphins playing a key role. Endorphins are neurotransmitters that act as natural mood elevators and pain relievers. The increased production of endorphins during and after strength training contributes to a sense of well-being, reduced feelings of stress, and an overall improvement in mood.

Reduction of Anxiety and Depression Symptoms:

Regular strength training has shown promising results in reducing symptoms of anxiety and depression. The physiological and psychological benefits of strength training, including the release of neurotransmitters like serotonin and the alleviation of cortisol levels, contribute to the management of mood disorders. Strength training is often recommended as a complementary intervention alongside traditional treatments for anxiety and depression.

Cognitive Function and Memory Improvement:

Strength training has cognitive benefits that extend to improved cognitive function and memory. Research suggests that resistance exercise can positively impact executive functions, such as attention, working memory, and problem-solving skills. This cognitive enhancement can contribute to overall mental acuity and resilience.

Neuroplasticity and Brain Health:

Strength training promotes neuroplasticity, the brain's ability to reorganize and form new neural connections. This is particularly important for maintaining brain health and preventing cognitive decline. Engaging in regular strength training has been associated with a protective effect against age-related cognitive decline and neurodegenerative diseases.

Stress Reduction and Cortisol Regulation:

Strength training helps regulate cortisol levels, the hormone associated with stress. By engaging in regular physical activity, individuals can manage and reduce chronic stress, preventing the negative impact of prolonged cortisol elevation on mental health. The combination of physical exertion, improved hormonal balance, and the sense of accomplishment from strength training contributes to stress reduction.

Improved Sleep Quality:
Sleep and mental health are intricately linked. Strength training has been shown to improve sleep quality, leading to better mental and emotional well-being. Quality sleep is essential for mood regulation, cognitive function, and overall mental health. The physical exertion and hormonal changes induced by strength training contribute to more restful sleep.

Enhanced Self-Esteem and Confidence:
Achieving strength training goals, whether it's lifting heavier weights or mastering challenging exercises, contributes to a sense of accomplishment and self-efficacy. This boost in self-esteem and confidence positively influences overall mental health. Feeling capable and strong can translate into a more

positive self-image and resilience in the face of life's challenges.

Social Interaction and Support:
Strength training can be a social activity, fostering connections with others who share similar fitness goals. Social interaction and support are crucial components of mental health. Building relationships within a fitness community or working out with a partner provides a sense of belonging and contributes to positive mood and emotional well-being.

Stress Resilience and Coping Mechanisms:
Engaging in regular strength training builds physical and mental resilience. The discipline, consistency, and determination required for strength training serve as valuable coping mechanisms for managing stress and adversity. Individuals who practice strength training develop a mindset of resilience that extends beyond the gym, positively influencing their ability to cope with life's challenges.

Long-Term Mental Health Benefits:

The cumulative effects of strength training, when integrated into a long-term routine, contribute to sustained mental health benefits. Regular exercise becomes a proactive strategy for managing mood, stress, and cognitive function throughout one's life, promoting overall mental well-being.

In conclusion, strength training has a multifaceted impact on mental health, encompassing mood enhancement, cognitive benefits, stress reduction, and overall psychological well-being. Incorporating strength training into a holistic approach to mental health can be a powerful and sustainable strategy for individuals seeking to optimize their emotional and cognitive resilience.

CHAPTER FIVE

The relationship between strength training and the prevention of chronic diseases

Research has consistently demonstrated a strong relationship between strength training and the prevention of various chronic diseases. Engaging in regular strength training exercises has been associated with numerous health benefits that contribute to the prevention, management, and reduction of the risk of chronic diseases. Here's an overview on the relationship between strength training and the prevention of specific chronic diseases:

Type 2 Diabetes

Research Findings: Numerous studies have shown that strength training can improve insulin sensitivity and glycemic control, which are crucial factors in preventing and managing type 2 diabetes. A meta-analysis published in the "Journal of the American Medical Association" found that resistance training was associated with a significant reduction in the risk of developing type 2 diabetes.

Cardiovascular Disease:

Research Findings: Strength training has cardiovascular benefits, including improvements in blood pressure, lipid profile, and overall heart health. A systematic review and meta-analysis published in "Sports Medicine" indicated that resistance training was associated with a significant reduction in blood pressure, particularly in individuals with hypertension. Strength training has also been shown to improve cardiovascular risk factors, such as reducing LDL cholesterol and increasing HDL cholesterol.

Osteoporosis:

Research Findings: Resistance training is effective in promoting bone health and reducing the risk of osteoporosis. Research published in the "Journal of Bone and Mineral Research" suggests that strength training can increase bone mineral density, particularly in postmenopausal women. The mechanical stress placed on bones during resistance exercises stimulates bone formation and helps prevent bone loss associated with aging.

Arthritis:

Research Findings: Strength training has been shown to be beneficial for individuals with arthritis by improving joint function, reducing pain, and enhancing overall quality of life. A study published in "Arthritis & Rheumatism" found that a 12-week resistance training program led to significant improvements in physical function and reduced symptoms in individuals with knee osteoarthritis.

Depression and Anxiety:

Research Findings: Strength training has positive effects on mental health, including the prevention and management of depression and anxiety. A meta-analysis published in "JAMA Psychiatry" concluded that resistance exercise significantly reduced symptoms of depression. The psychological benefits of strength training, such as the release of endorphins and improved self-esteem, contribute to its role in mental health.

Cancer:

Research Findings: Emerging evidence suggests that strength training may have protective effects against certain types of cancer. While more research is needed in this area, some studies have shown associations between resistance training and a lower risk of developing breast and colon cancer. Additionally, strength training has been found to improve the quality of life and physical function in cancer survivors.

Chronic Kidney Disease:

Research Findings: Strength training has been studied as a potential intervention for individuals with chronic kidney disease (CKD). Research published in the "American Journal of Kidney Diseases" suggests that resistance training may improve muscle strength, physical function, and quality of life in individuals with CKD. However, more research is needed to establish specific guidelines for strength training in this population.

Neurological Disorders:
Research Findings: Strength training has shown promise in benefiting individuals with neurological disorders such as Parkinson's disease. Research published in "Neurorehabilitation and Neural Repair" indicates that resistance training can improve motor function,

strength, and quality of life in individuals with Parkinson's disease. Similar benefits have been observed in other neurological conditions.

In summary, research consistently supports the positive impact of strength training on the prevention and management of various chronic diseases. The benefits extend beyond musculoskeletal health to encompass metabolic, cardiovascular, mental, and neurological well-being. Incorporating regular strength training into a comprehensive health and fitness routine is a valuable strategy for promoting overall health and reducing the risk of chronic diseases. Individuals should consult with healthcare professionals or fitness experts to develop personalized strength training programs, especially if they have existing health conditions.

How strength training contribute to cardiovascular health and diabetes prevention.

Strength training, traditionally associated with building muscle and strength, plays a crucial role in promoting cardiovascular health and preventing the onset of type 2 diabetes. While aerobic exercise like running or cycling is commonly recommended for cardiovascular benefits, emerging research highlights the significant positive impact of strength training on heart health and diabetes prevention. Here's how strength training contributes to cardiovascular health and diabetes prevention:

Cardiovascular Health:

Blood Pressure Regulation:

Strength training has been shown to contribute to the regulation of blood pressure. Regular resistance exercise can lead to decreases in both systolic and diastolic blood pressure, particularly beneficial for individuals with hypertension. This effect is thought to be a result of improved blood vessel function and reduced stiffness.

Improvement in Lipid Profile:

Strength training has a positive impact on lipid metabolism, leading to improvements in the lipid profile. Studies have demonstrated reductions in total cholesterol, LDL cholesterol (the "bad" cholesterol), and triglycerides, as well as increases in HDL cholesterol (the "good" cholesterol) in response to regular resistance exercise.

Enhanced Endothelial Function:

Endothelial function refers to the health of the inner lining of blood vessels. Strength training has been associated with improved endothelial function, which is vital for maintaining healthy blood vessels. This improvement contributes to better blood flow, reduced risk of atherosclerosis, and overall cardiovascular health.

Reduced Arterial Stiffness:

Arterial stiffness is a marker of vascular health and is linked to an increased risk of cardiovascular events. Strength training has been shown to reduce arterial stiffness, contributing to better elasticity in blood vessels. This reduction in stiffness helps lower the workload on the heart and improves overall cardiovascular function.

Increased Cardiac Output:

Strength training results in increased cardiac output, the amount of blood the heart pumps per minute. This adaptation is beneficial for cardiovascular health as it enhances the heart's efficiency in delivering oxygen and nutrients to the body's tissues. Improved cardiac output is associated with better cardiovascular endurance.

Metabolic syndrome is a cluster of conditions that increase the risk of heart disease, stroke, and type 2 diabetes. Strength training has been shown to have a positive impact on metabolic syndrome by addressing risk factors such as abdominal obesity, insulin resistance, and high blood pressure.

✓ *Diabetes Prevention:*

Improved Insulin Sensitivity:

Insulin sensitivity is a key factor in preventing type 2 diabetes. Strength training has been consistently linked to improvements in insulin sensitivity, allowing cells to more effectively respond to insulin and regulate blood sugar levels. This is particularly important in reducing the risk of insulin resistance, a precursor to diabetes.

Enhanced Glucose Metabolism:

Strength training positively influences glucose metabolism by promoting the uptake of glucose by muscle cells. This helps maintain blood sugar levels within a healthy range. Studies have shown that individuals engaging in regular resistance exercise exhibit better postprandial (after-meal) glucose control.

Body Composition and Weight Management:

Strength training contributes to improvements in body composition, including increased lean muscle mass and reduced body fat. This shift in body composition is beneficial for preventing obesity, a major risk factor for type 2 diabetes. Maintaining a healthy weight through strength training supports overall metabolic health.

Reduced Abdominal Fat:

Abdominal fat, particularly visceral fat, is strongly associated with an increased risk of type 2 diabetes. Strength training has been shown to reduce abdominal fat, which is critical for diabetes prevention. Targeting visceral fat through resistance exercise contributes to a healthier metabolic profile.

Long-Term Maintenance of Muscle Mass:

As individuals age, there is a natural tendency to lose muscle mass, which can contribute to insulin resistance. Strength training is essential for the long-term maintenance of muscle mass, helping to preserve metabolic health and prevent age-related declines in insulin sensitivity.

Improved Blood Sugar Control:

Strength training, when combined with aerobic exercise, has been found to be effective in improving overall blood sugar control. This combined approach is often recommended for individuals at risk of or managing type 2 diabetes, providing comprehensive benefits for metabolic health.

In conclusion, strength training is a versatile and effective strategy for promoting cardiovascular health and preventing type 2 diabetes. Its impact extends beyond building muscle to include improvements in blood pressure, lipid profile, endothelial function, and insulin sensitivity. Incorporating strength training into a well-rounded fitness routine, along with other healthy lifestyle habits, is a powerful approach to maintaining cardiovascular health and reducing the risk of chronic metabolic conditions. Individuals should consult with healthcare professionals or fitness experts to develop personalized strength training programs, especially if they have existing health conditions.

CHAPTER SIX

How strength training shapes and tones the body.

Strength training plays a role in body composition by promoting fat loss and lean muscle gain. As muscle mass increases, the body's metabolism is boosted, leading to an increase in calorie expenditure, both during and after workouts. This contributes to a reduction in body fat percentage, revealing the sculpted and toned appearance of the muscles beneath.

Definition and Muscle Visibility:

Strength training enhances muscle definition by targeting specific muscle groups. Exercises such as bicep curls, tricep dips, and leg presses isolate and engage specific muscles, creating more pronounced contours. As body fat decreases and muscle mass increases, the visibility of these defined muscle groups improves, contributing to a toned physique.

Functional Strength:

Beyond aesthetics, strength training builds functional strength, improving the body's ability to perform everyday activities. Compound exercises, such as squats and deadlifts, engage multiple muscle groups simultaneously, promoting overall functional fitness. This combination of strength and functionality contributes to a well-toned and capable body.

Increased Muscle Density:

Strength training not only increases muscle size but also enhances muscle density. This is the result of improvements in muscle quality, including increased protein synthesis and structural adaptations. The denser and firmer appearance of the muscles adds to the overall toning effect.

Spot Reduction:

While spot reduction (losing fat from a specific area through exercise targeting that area) is a debated concept, strength training can contribute to localized fat loss. By focusing on specific muscle groups, strength training promotes localized metabolism, potentially reducing fat in targeted areas and enhancing the toning effect.

Improved Posture and Alignment:

Strength training exercises often involve core engagement and stabilization, leading to improved posture and body alignment. A strong and well-supported core contributes to a more upright and sculpted appearance. Exercises that target the back, shoulders, and core, such as rows and planks, are particularly effective in enhancing posture.

Balanced Muscle Development:

A well-designed strength training program ensures balanced muscle development. Targeting opposing muscle groups, such as the quadriceps and hamstrings, or the chest and back, helps prevent muscle imbalances. Balanced development contributes to a symmetrical and aesthetically pleasing physique.

Reduction of Body Fluctuations:

Strength training helps reduce body fluctuations by building a stable foundation of lean muscle mass. This stability contributes to a more consistent and toned appearance, minimizing fluctuations caused by changes in body composition.

Increased Muscle Definition at Any Age:

Strength training is beneficial for individuals of all ages, and its effects on muscle definition are not limited to younger populations. Older adults can also experience increased muscle definition and toning through consistent strength training, contributing to improved functionality and quality of life.

In summary, strength training shapes and tones the body by promoting muscle hypertrophy, reducing body fat, enhancing definition, and improving overall body composition. A well-rounded strength training program, combined with proper nutrition and recovery, is key to achieving a sculpted and toned physique. Individuals should tailor their strength training routines to their specific goals and fitness levels, and consult with fitness professionals for guidance and support.

Examples of exercises that target specific muscle groups for a well-rounded physique.

A well-rounded strength training program should target various muscle groups to promote balanced development and overall muscular fitness. Incorporating exercises that engage different parts of the body ensures comprehensive strength and enhances both aesthetics and functionality. Here are examples of exercises that target specific muscle groups for a well-rounded physique:

✓ *Quadriceps (Front of Thighs):*

Exercise: Barbell Back Squat

How to: Stand with feet shoulder-width apart, a barbell across your upper back. Lower your body by bending at the hips and knees, keeping your back straight. Descend until your thighs are parallel to the ground, then push back up to the starting position.

✓ *Hamstrings (Back of Thighs):*

Exercise: Romanian Deadlift

How to: Hold a barbell with an overhand grip, hands shoulder-width apart. Hinge at the hips, keeping the back straight, and lower the barbell towards the floor. Keep a slight bend in the knees. Return to the starting position by driving the hips forward.

Exercise: Barbell Hip Thrust

How to: Sit on the ground with a barbell across your hips. Roll the barbell towards you, so it sits just above your hips. Plant your feet firmly and lift your hips towards the ceiling, squeezing your glutes at the top. Lower back down and repeat.

✓ *Chest (Pectoral Muscles):*

Exercise: Barbell Bench Press

How to: Lie on a flat bench with a barbell at chest height. Grip the bar with hands slightly wider than shoulder-width apart. Lower the bar to your chest, then push it back up to the starting position.

✓ *Back (Latissimus Dorsi and Rhomboids):*

Exercise: Bent Over Barbell Row

How to: Stand with a barbell in front of you, feet shoulder-width apart. Bend at the hips, keeping your back straight, and grip the barbell with hands slightly wider than shoulder-width. Pull the barbell towards your lower chest, then lower it back down.

✓ *Shoulders (Deltoid Muscles):*

Exercise: Standing Dumbbell Shoulder Press

How to: Hold a dumbbell in each hand at shoulder height. Press the dumbbells overhead, fully extending your arms. Lower them back to shoulder height and repeat.

✓ *Biceps (Biceps Brachii):*

Exercise: Barbell Bicep Curl

How to: Stand with a barbell in front of you, palms facing forward. Keep your elbows close to your body as you curl the barbell towards your shoulders. Lower it back down and repeat.

✓ *Triceps (Triceps Brachii):*

Exercise: Tricep Dips

How to: Sit on a bench or parallel bars with your hands placed next to your hips. Lower your body by bending your elbows until your upper arms are parallel to the ground. Push back up to the starting position.

✓ *Core (Abdominals and Obliques):*

Exercise: Plank

How to: Get into a push-up position, but with your weight on your forearms. Keep your body in a straight line from head to heels, engaging your core muscles. Hold the position for as long as possible.

✓ *Calves (Gastrocnemius and Soleus):*

Exercise: Standing Calf Raise

How to: Stand with feet hip-width apart, and lift your heels off the ground by pushing through the balls of your feet. Lower your heels back down and repeat.

✓ *Full Body (Compound Exercise):*

Exercise: Deadlift

How to: Stand with feet hip-width apart, a barbell in front of you. Bend at the hips and knees to lower your body and grip the barbell. Lift the barbell by extending your hips and knees, keeping your back straight.

Exercise: High-Intensity Interval Training (HIIT)

How to: Incorporate short bursts of intense exercise (e.g., sprinting, jumping jacks) followed by periods of rest or lower intensity. HIIT can enhance cardiovascular fitness and burn additional calories.

Remember to start with a weight that allows you to maintain proper form and gradually progress as your strength increases. It's also essential to warm up before strength training and cool down afterward to prevent injuries and promote flexibility. If you're new to strength training or have any health concerns, consider consulting with a fitness professional or healthcare provider to design a program tailored to your needs.

CHAPTER SEVEN

How strength training improves functional fitness.

Strength training is a key component of improving functional fitness, which involves enhancing the body's ability to perform everyday activities with efficiency, ease, and reduced risk of injury. Unlike isolated exercises that target individual muscles, strength training focuses on compound movements that engage multiple muscle groups simultaneously. Here's an illustration of how strength training improves functional fitness:

Enhanced Muscle Strength:

Illustration: Imagine trying to carry a heavy bag of groceries up a flight of stairs. With increased muscle strength from strength training, your muscles can generate more force, making tasks like carrying groceries or lifting objects much easier and less fatiguing.

Improved Joint Stability:

Illustration: Consider the act of bending down to tie your shoelaces. Strength training stabilizes the joints by strengthening the muscles around them. This added stability allows for better control and reduces the risk of joint-related injuries during daily activities.

Increased Bone Density:

Illustration: Picture walking or running on uneven surfaces. Strength training contributes to increased bone density, providing better support and protection against fractures or injuries related to impact or falls.

Functional Movement Patterns:

Illustration: Think about the motion of squatting down to pick something up from the ground. Strength training emphasizes functional movement patterns like squats, lunges, and deadlifts, making these activities more efficient and reducing the risk of injury during daily tasks.

Enhanced Balance and Coordination:

Illustration: Imagine navigating through a crowded area or maintaining balance while carrying a tray. Strength training improves balance and coordination by activating stabilizing muscles and promoting better control over body movements.

Improved Posture:

Illustration: Envision sitting at a desk for an extended period. Strength training, especially exercises targeting the core and back muscles, helps improve posture. This not only reduces the risk of developing musculoskeletal issues but also enhances comfort during prolonged periods of sitting or standing.

Functional Core Strength:

Illustration: Consider the act of bending and twisting to reach for an item. Strength training, including core exercises, enhances functional core strength, which is crucial for maintaining spinal alignment and supporting various movements in daily life.

Efficient Energy Expenditure:

Illustration: Picture climbing a set of stairs effortlessly. Strength training improves muscular endurance, allowing you to perform activities with less fatigue and more efficient energy expenditure.

Injury Prevention:

Illustration: Imagine stepping off a curb without fear of tripping. Strength training, by addressing muscular imbalances and weaknesses, reduces the risk of falls and injuries associated with everyday movements.

Functional Adaptations to Aging:

Illustration: Think about the challenges of getting up from a chair as you age. Strength training helps maintain muscle mass, strength, and power, providing functional adaptations that support independent living and mobility in older adults.

Increased Range of Motion:

Illustration: Visualize reaching for an item on a high shelf. Strength training, combined with flexibility exercises, improves joint mobility and increases the range of motion, making such tasks more accessible and reducing the risk of strains.

Better Proprioception:

Illustration: Consider navigating a dimly lit room. Strength training enhances proprioception, the body's awareness of its position in space, improving your ability to move confidently and efficiently, even in challenging environments.

Including a well-rounded strength training program into your fitness routine helps you build a foundation of functional fitness. The benefits extend beyond the gym, positively impacting your ability to perform daily activities with ease, reducing the risk of injury, and enhancing overall quality of life. Always consult with a fitness professional or healthcare provider before starting a new exercise program, especially if you have specific health considerations.

Examples of some exercises that mimic everyday activities for practical benefits.

Doing some of the exercises that mimic everyday activities is an effective way to enhance functional fitness. These movements not only improve strength but also translate directly into improved performance in daily tasks. Here are examples of exercises that mimic everyday activities for practical benefits:

✓ *Squats*:

Everyday Activity: Sitting down and standing up from a chair or toilet.

Exercise: Bodyweight Squat or Goblet Squat

How to: Stand with feet shoulder-width apart, lower your body by bending at the hips and knees, and then push back up to the starting position.

✓ *Lunges*:

Everyday Activity: Walking, ascending or descending stairs.

Exercise: Forward or Reverse Lunges

How to: Take a step forward or backward, lower your body until both knees are bent at a 90-degree angle, then return to the starting position.

✓ *Deadlifts*:

Everyday Activity: Lifting objects from the ground (e.g., groceries, laundry).

Exercise: Conventional or Romanian Deadlift

How to: With a barbell or dumbbells, hinge at the hips while keeping your back straight, lowering the weight towards the ground, then return to an upright position.

✓ *Push-Ups:*

Everyday Activity: Pushing yourself up from a surface (e.g., getting up from the ground).

Exercise: Standard or Modified Push-Ups

How to: Begin in a plank position, lower your body by bending your elbows, then push back up to the starting position.

✓ *Pull-Ups or Lat Pulldowns:*

Everyday Activity: Pulling or lifting objects towards you.

Exercise: Pull-Ups or Lat Pulldowns

How to: Grip a bar overhead, pull your body up, or pull the bar down towards your chest, engaging your back muscles.

✓ *Farmers Walk:*

Everyday Activity: Carrying heavy bags or groceries.

Exercise: Farmers Walk

How to: Hold a weight (dumbbells or kettlebells) in each hand, maintain an upright posture, and walk a certain distance or for a specific duration.

✓ *Step-Ups:*

Everyday Activity: Climbing stairs or stepping onto elevated surfaces.

Exercise: Step-Ups

How to: Step onto a sturdy surface, ensuring your entire foot is on the surface, then step back down.

✓ *Planks*:

Everyday Activity: Maintaining a stable and strong core during various movements.

Exercise: Front Plank or Side Plank
How to: Hold a plank position, either facing the ground or on your side, engaging your core muscles.

✓ *Woodchopper (Medicine Ball or Cable):*
Everyday Activity: Rotational movements, such as reaching for items.

Exercise: Woodchopper
How to: Using a medicine ball or cable machine, simulate a chopping motion across your body, engaging your core and oblique muscles.

✓ *Kettlebell Swings:*
Everyday Activity: Lifting and swinging motions (e.g., picking up a child or swinging a bag).

Exercise: Kettlebell Swing
How to: With a kettlebell between your legs, hinge at the hips and swing the kettlebell forward, using the power generated from your hips.

✓ *Seated Row:*

Everyday Activity: Pulling or rowing motions, such as closing a car door.

Exercise: Seated Cable Row

How to: Sit at a cable row machine, grasp the handle, and pull it towards you, squeezing your shoulder blades together.

✓ *Balancing Exercises:*

Everyday Activity: Maintaining balance during various activities.

Exercise: Single-Leg Stance or Bosu Ball Exercises

How to: Stand on one leg or on an unstable surface, engaging your core and lower body muscles to maintain balance.

Incorporating these functional exercises into your fitness routine helps build strength, stability, and mobility that directly transfer to improved performance in everyday activities. Always prioritize proper form and, if needed, consult with a fitness professional to tailor exercises to your specific needs and abilities.

CHAPTER EIGHT

CUSTOMIZED WORKOUTS FOR WOMEN

The importance of tailoring strength training routines for individual needs.

Tailoring strength training routines to individual needs is crucial for maximizing effectiveness, safety, and long-term adherence. People have unique goals, fitness levels, health considerations, and preferences, and a one-size-fits-all approach may not address these individual factors adequately. Here's a discussion on the importance of customizing strength training routines:

Achieving Personal Goals:

Importance: Individuals pursue strength training for various reasons, including muscle building, fat loss, improved athletic performance, or rehabilitation. Tailoring a routine ensures that the exercises and intensity align with specific goals, promoting more targeted and efficient progress.

Addressing Fitness Levels:

Importance: Fitness levels vary widely among individuals, and a routine that is too challenging or too easy can be demotivating or potentially harmful. Customizing the intensity, volume, and complexity of exercises allows for gradual progression based on the individual's current fitness level.

Considering Health and Medical Factors:

Importance: Medical conditions, injuries, or specific health concerns influence the type and intensity of exercises that are suitable. A tailored routine considers these factors, ensuring that individuals can engage in strength training safely and without exacerbating existing health issues.

Enhancing Motivation and Adherence:

Importance: Personalized programs are more likely to align with an individual's preferences and interests. Enjoyable and engaging routines increase motivation and adherence, making it more likely for individuals to stick with their strength training over the long term.

Optimizing Time and Resources:

Importance: Tailoring a routine takes into account time constraints, available equipment, and the individual's lifestyle. An efficient and practical plan that fits into daily life encourages consistency and adherence to the strength training program.

Balancing Strength and Flexibility:

Importance: Strength training should not neglect flexibility. Tailored programs can incorporate a balance of strength and flexibility exercises, addressing the importance of maintaining a full range of motion and preventing injuries related to muscle imbalances.

Preventing Overtraining and Burnout:

Importance: Individual recovery capacity varies, and pushing too hard without adequate rest can lead to overtraining and burnout. Customizing the frequency and intensity of workouts ensures an appropriate balance between challenging the body and allowing for sufficient recovery.

Adapting to Age and Life Stage:

Importance: Age-related factors, such as muscle loss and joint health, influence the ideal strength training routine. Customizing exercises to accommodate these factors allows for safe and effective training throughout different life stages.

Accommodating Preferences and Enjoyment:

Importance: Everyone has different preferences regarding exercise types, environments, and formats. Tailoring a routine to align with these preferences fosters a positive attitude towards strength training, making it more enjoyable and sustainable.

Individualizing Progression Strategies:

Importance: Progression is a key aspect of strength training success. Tailoring the rate of progression, adding variety, and adjusting the difficulty of exercises ensures that individuals are continually challenged without risking injury or plateauing.

Providing Education and Guidance:

Importance: Customized routines should be accompanied by education and guidance. Understanding the purpose of exercises, proper form, and the overall structure of the program empowers individuals to take ownership of their fitness journey.

Adapting to Changing Circumstances:

Importance: Life circumstances, such as changes in work schedules, family responsibilities, or health status, may require adjustments to the strength training routine. Personalization allows for ongoing adaptation to changing circumstances.

In conclusion, the importance of tailoring strength training routines for individual needs cannot be overstated. Whether working with a fitness professional or designing a program independently, individuals should consider their unique goals, fitness levels, health conditions, and preferences. A personalized approach ensures that strength training becomes a sustainable and enjoyable part of an individual's lifestyle, leading to improved fitness, health, and overall well-being.

Guidance on selecting the right exercises and adjusting intensity.

Designing a strength training program tailored to women involves considering individual goals, fitness levels, preferences, and any specific considerations. Here's guidance on selecting the right exercises and adjusting intensity for women:

Define Your Goals:

- *Guidance*: Clarify your fitness goals. Whether it's building strength, toning muscles, improving overall health, or addressing specific concerns (e.g., bone density, postpartum recovery), your goals will shape exercise selection and intensity.

Assess Your Fitness Level:

- *Guidance*: Evaluate your current fitness level objectively. Choose exercises that align with your abilities. Beginners should start with foundational movements, while more advanced individuals can incorporate a broader range of exercises.

Include Full-Body Compound Movements:

- *Guidance*: Prioritize compound exercises that engage multiple muscle groups simultaneously. Examples include squats, deadlifts, lunges, bench presses, and rows. These movements efficiently target multiple muscle groups and boost overall strength.

Incorporate Functional Movements:

- *Guidance*: Include exercises that mimic real-life movements. Functional movements enhance overall functionality, making daily activities more manageable. Examples include squats, lunges, and kettlebell swings.

Diversify Your Routine:

- *Guidance*: Add variety to your workouts. Include exercises that target different muscle groups and movement patterns. This not only prevents boredom but also ensures comprehensive muscle development.

Consider Equipment Availability:

- *Guidance*: Adapt your exercises based on available equipment. Whether using free weights, machines, resistance bands, or bodyweight, choose exercises that fit your resources and preferences.

Balance Cardiovascular and Strength Training:

- *Guidance*: Integrate cardiovascular exercises with strength training. This combination offers holistic fitness benefits, including improved heart health, endurance, and weight management.

Adjust for Individual Needs:

- *Guidance*: Modify exercises based on individual needs or restrictions. For instance, consider low-impact variations if you have joint concerns or seek guidance from fitness professionals for personalized adjustments.

Remember that personalization is key when designing a strength training program for women. Consider your preferences, individual needs, and lifestyle to create a sustainable and enjoyable fitness routine. Always consult with healthcare professionals or fitness experts, especially if you have specific health considerations or concerns.

CHAPTER NINE

The psychological aspect of feeling strong and capable.

Feeling strong and capable, both physically and mentally, has profound psychological benefits that extend beyond the physical realm. This sense of strength contributes significantly to an individual's overall well-being and mental health. Here's an exploration of the psychological aspects of feeling strong and capable:

Enhanced Self-Efficacy:

Explanation: Achieving strength-related goals fosters a sense of self-efficacy — the belief in one's ability to succeed in specific situations. Overcoming physical challenges translates into confidence in tackling various life challenges.

Increased Confidence and Self-esteem:

Explanation: **Strength gains and physical accomplishments directly impact self-esteem. As individuals see progress in their strength training journey, they often experience an enhanced sense of confidence, both in their physical abilities and their overall self-worth.**

Empowerment and Control:

Explanation: **Strength training provides a tangible way to exert control over one's body and physical capabilities. The empowerment gained from mastering new exercises or lifting heavier weights can extend to a feeling of control in other aspects of life.**

Stress Reduction and Resilience:

Explanation: **Regular physical activity, including strength training, is associated with reduced stress levels. Feeling physically strong enhances resilience, providing individuals with a coping mechanism to better navigate stressors and challenges.**

Mood Enhancement:

Explanation: **Exercise, particularly strength training, triggers the release of endorphins, the body's natural mood elevators. The positive feelings associated with exercise contribute to an improved overall mood and** can serve as a natural antidote to feelings of anxiety or depression.

Body Positivity and Acceptance:

Explanation: Strength training promotes a positive relationship with one's body. Rather than focusing solely on appearance, individuals shift their perspective to what their bodies can do. This shift can foster body acceptance and a more positive body image.

Improved Mental Resilience:

Explanation: Overcoming physical challenges in strength training builds mental resilience. This resilience can translate into increased capacity to navigate life's obstacles, bounce back from setbacks, and maintain a positive mindset.

Positive Feedback Loop:

Explanation: Progress in strength training creates a positive feedback loop. As individuals see improvements in their physical capabilities, they are motivated to continue their efforts, reinforcing a cycle of positive reinforcement and accomplishment.

Sense of Competence:

Explanation: Mastering complex movements and achieving fitness goals instills a sense of competence.

This feeling of competence extends beyond the gym, influencing how individuals approach tasks and challenges in various areas of life.

CHAPTER TEN

STORIES OF WOMEN WHO HAVE EXPERIENCED INCREASED CONFIDENCE THROUGH STRENGTH TRAINING.

Certainly! Here are a few inspirational stories of women who have experienced increased confidence through strength training:

Molly Galbraith - Co-Founder of Girls Gone Strong:

Molly Galbraith, co-founder of Girls Gone Strong, struggled with body image issues and societal expectations. Through strength training, she found a way to appreciate her body for its capabilities rather than its appearance. Molly's journey not only transformed her physically but also led her to create a community empowering women in strength and fitness.

Arlene Semeco - Powerlifter and Coach:

Story: Arlene Semeco, a powerlifter and coach, discovered strength training after facing challenges with body image and self-esteem. As she progressed in lifting heavier weights, Arlene noticed a significant shift in her confidence. Embracing her strength not only transformed her physical self but also empowered her mentally.

Anna Victoria - Fitness Influencer:

Story: Anna Victoria, a fitness influencer, initially focused on aesthetics but later shifted her mindset towards strength and performance. Through her strength training journey, she gained a newfound appreciation for her body's capabilities. Anna encourages women to prioritize strength and health over societal beauty standards.

Stephanie Buttermore - YouTuber and PhD:

Story: Stephanie Buttermore, a YouTuber and PhD, went through a personal transformation by embracing a strength-focused approach to fitness. She moved away from restrictive eating and excessive cardio, focusing instead on strength training. Stephanie's journey is a testament to the mental and physical benefits of adopting a strength-centric mindset.

Katie Crewe - Fitness Trainer and Influencer:

Story: Katie Crewe, a fitness trainer and influencer, discovered strength training as a means to overcome her insecurities. Through consistent training, Katie not only built physical strength but also gained mental resilience. She emphasizes the importance of embracing one's journey and focusing on progress rather than perfection.

Meghan Callaway - Strength Coach:

Story: Meghan Callaway, a strength coach, shares her journey of overcoming body image issues and finding confidence through strength training. As she became stronger physically, Meghan's mindset evolved, and she now encourages women to pursue strength for the empowerment it brings.

Lindsay Cappotelli - Powerlifter and Coach:

Story: Lindsay Cappotelli, a powerlifter and coach, discovered strength training as a way to challenge herself physically and mentally. As she achieved new milestones in lifting, Lindsay's confidence soared. She advocates for women to step into the weight room with confidence and embrace their strength.

Lizzo - Musician and Body Positivity Advocate:

Story: Lizzo, a Grammy-winning musician, incorporates strength training into her routine as part of her journey towards body positivity. She shares her workouts on social media, emphasizing the joy and empowerment that comes from moving and strengthening her body.

Jen Sinkler - Strength Coach and Writer:

Story: Jen Sinkler, a strength coach and writer, discovered the transformative power of strength training both for her body and mind. Her journey showcases how strength can be a source of empowerment, breaking away from societal expectations and fostering self-confidence.

These stories illustrate the diverse ways in which women have found empowerment, confidence, and a positive body image through strength training. The shift from aesthetics-focused goals to celebrating what their bodies can do has been a common thread in these journeys, emphasizing the holistic benefits of strength training on mental well-being.

CHAPTER ELEVEN

SOCIAL AND COMMUNITY ASPECTS: The social benefits of group strength training classes.

Group strength training classes offer numerous social benefits that go beyond the physical aspects of fitness. Here are some highlights of the social benefits of participating in group strength training classes:

Built-In Support System:

Explanation: Group classes create a sense of community, providing participants with a built-in support system. Working out alongside others fosters camaraderie and mutual encouragement, creating a positive and motivating atmosphere.

Motivation and Accountability:

Explanation: The group setting adds a layer of accountability. Knowing that others are expecting your presence can be a powerful motivator to attend classes regularly. This shared commitment encourages consistency in participants' fitness routines.

Sense of Belonging:

Explanation: Group classes offer a sense of belonging and inclusion. Participants become part of a fitness community where everyone shares a common goal of improving strength and overall well-being. This sense of belonging enhances the overall fitness experience.

Social Interaction:

Explanation: Group strength training classes provide opportunities for social interaction. Whether it's chatting before or after class, sharing workout tips, or celebrating achievements together, the social component adds an enjoyable dimension to the exercise routine.

Variety of Perspectives:

Explanation: Group classes attract individuals with diverse backgrounds, fitness levels, and experiences. This diversity brings a variety of perspectives and insights into the fitness journey, creating a rich environment for learning and personal growth.

Increased Adherence to Exercise:

Explanation: The social aspect of group classes increases adherence to exercise. Knowing that others are expecting you can make it more likely for participants to prioritize and maintain their fitness routines, leading to long-term health benefits.

Friendly Competition:

Explanation: A bit of friendly competition within the group can be a positive motivator. Whether it's lifting heavier weights, completing more reps, or achieving personal bests, the collective energy of the group can drive individuals to push their limits.

Shared Challenges and Triumphs:

Explanation: Participants in group strength training classes share common challenges and triumphs. Whether it's conquering a difficult exercise or reaching a fitness milestone, the shared experiences create a sense of unity and shared accomplishment.

Expert Guidance and Support:

Explanation: Instructors in group classes provide expert guidance and support. Participants benefit from the knowledge and encouragement of a trained professional, ensuring they perform exercises correctly and safely.

In summary, the social benefits of group strength training classes create a supportive and motivating environment that enhances the overall fitness experience. The sense of community, shared goals, and positive interactions contribute to not only physical health but also emotional well-being and a sense of connection with others.

The sense of community and support that can be found in strength training environments.

Strength training environments, whether they be in traditional gyms, specialized fitness centers, or community-based workout groups, often foster a strong sense of community and support among participants. This sense of camaraderie and shared goals contributes significantly to the overall positive experience of engaging in strength training. Here are some key aspects that contribute to the sense of community in strength training environments:

Shared Goals and Aspirations:

Strength training environments attract individuals with similar fitness goals, such as building muscle, improving strength, or enhancing overall fitness.

Participants often share a common commitment to self-improvement and a dedication to achieving their personal fitness objectives.

Encouragement and Motivation:

The process of lifting weights or engaging in resistance training can be challenging, and having a supportive community around can provide motivation during difficult workouts.

Fellow participants and trainers often offer words of encouragement, celebrate achievements, and provide the push needed to overcome obstacles.

Knowledge Sharing:

Strength training environments are conducive to the exchange of knowledge and expertise.

Experienced individuals often share tips, techniques, and insights with newcomers, creating a learning environment that benefits participants of all skill levels.

Accountability:

The presence of a supportive community fosters a sense of accountability. Knowing that others are aware of your fitness goals can encourage consistency and dedication to the training regimen.

Group workouts or training partners can also create a sense of responsibility, as individuals are less

CHAPTER TWELVE

In conclusion, strength exercise for women offers multifaceted benefits that extend far beyond physical appearance. Through resistance training, women can significantly enhance their overall health and well-being. The evidence presented underscores the importance of strength training as a means to promote bone density, reduce the risk of osteoporosis, and mitigate the effects of aging-related muscle loss. Additionally, the psychological advantages cannot be overstated, with strength training demonstrating its efficacy in reducing stress, anxiety, and depression while enhancing self-esteem and confidence.

Furthermore, debunking myths surrounding strength training for women is crucial in encouraging participation and dispelling fears of becoming "bulky." The research indicates that women are physiologically predisposed to build lean muscle mass rather than excessive bulk, emphasizing the empowerment and control they can achieve over their bodies through structured resistance training programs.

Moreover, the inclusivity of strength training accommodates various fitness levels and goals, allowing women to tailor their workouts according to their preferences and capabilities. Whether aiming for increased strength, improved endurance, or enhanced functional fitness, women can find suitable exercises and progressions to meet their individual needs. Additionally, the social aspect of strength training, whether through group classes or online communities, fosters a sense of camaraderie and support, further motivating women to adhere to their exercise regimens. In essence, strength exercise for women is not merely about sculpting muscles or achieving a particular aesthetic; it's about cultivating resilience, fortifying the body against age-related decline, and fostering a positive mindset. By embracing strength training as an integral component of their wellness journey, women can unlock a wealth of physical and mental benefits, empowering them to lead healthier, more fulfilling lives.